Losing weight after 30

The makeover you deserve

Roxana Scurtu

Loosing weight in your 30's

DEDICATION

This book is dedicated to, my mother because she is the most perseverant and ambitious person I have ever known when it comes to weight loss.

Loosing weight in your 30's

Table of Contents

INTRODUCTION

I would like to start by thanking you for getting this book. If you are reading this, it's probably because you are tired of losing weight and gaining it back on. If you are looking for a permanent fix to your weight problems, you are in the right place. As women in our 30's, our metabolism doesn't assimilate and burn the calories as fast. It is also inconvenient to have to worry about dieting when we are so busy. This book will help you lose weight without making extreme sacrifices or sleeping at the gym. I wrote this book to help you make small changes to your lifestyle, which will have a big impact on your weight. I will not recommend the perfect diet but I will suggest some of the easiest and healthiest ones and it is your place to chose which one suits you better. Enjoy the book and get ready for a change.

Loosing weight in your 30's

CHAPTER 1 - DIETING AS A QUICK FIX

Taking care of one's health has always been a major concern for people. For the last 150 years or so, the Western world has come to realize that people should take care of their health in a rational and scientific way. Diet has been the most operative and functional area of concern as far as health care is concerned. As women in our 30s, out metabolic rate is slower and it get harder to lose weight.

Quite naturally, diet programs have gained enormous importance, and more and more people are becoming not only health conscious but diet conscious as well. Most of the people are concerned about the basic aspect of a diet program they just want to lose weight.

They say that weight loss does not start in the gym, it starts in the kitchen. The basic rule of weight loss is to burn more than your calorie intake - if you plan well enough for your diet, you may not need to work so hard at the gym.

Doing that means sacrificing bad eating habits, and usually, that's the difficult part and whats more challenging than that is to maintain it for a set period of time. As corporate people, we are often distracted by different factors like work stress, social obligations, tiredness - all these are usually what distract us from staying discipline to a strict diet - resorting to fast food because you just don't have enough time to prepare healthy food, you couldn't decline when your colleagues asked you to go to the bar, and you're so tired from work, you decided to just eat whatever unhealthy food you could find in your fridge.

If you are serious about losing weight, you should really consider changing habits and learn to force yourself to adhere to the diet plan. Fortunately planning healthy meals for your weight loss goals are not too difficult, but at the end of the day, as discussed is a matter of how much you stay in line with your plan.

Let me bring you right back to earth; save yourself from these claims. Anything that sounds too good to be true is probably is - rapid weight loss diets inclusive.

It's no news that Americans spend $33 billion every year on weight loss products, it is also no news that weight loss supplements and fad diets want a piece of that huge cake.

So, it's alright to believe these claims, after all, all you see are advert lines like "Lose 10 pounds in 10 Days" and "Drop one Dress Size today" plastered all over the internet.

Truth is, nothing like rapid weight loss diets exist and even if they do, they are unhealthy and can be counterproductive to your health and the weight is gained back on.

Now, you ask: Aren't rapid weight loss diets healthy? As far as I know, an A-listed celebrity once used it and never had a problem with it, what is then the problem?

A lot is wrong with these diets, I can tell you. But to quickly satisfy your curiosity, let's dive into this together. Any diet that promises drastic weight loss falls into any of the types below

Classes of Rapid Weight Loss Diets:

Very Low-Calorie Diets (VLCDs): These are supervised low-calorie diets based on researchers and studies on people that have used them and their effects on weight loss.

Starvation Diets: these diets promote detoxification through enemas or colonics. They promote a daily calorie intake of fewer than 1200 calories per day.

Diet Pills and Supplements: Just like the name, they are pills and supplements that promise to speed up weight loss by revving up your metabolism, burning fat in the process.

Creams and Devices: this type is the most dubious - lots of magic creams are out there that promise to replace exercise and healthy diet.

First, you need to know that marketers of these products make their claims freely - without any proof or any research to back them up.

The rapid weight loss diets worth considering is the VLCDs - the drastic reduction of calories - but even at that, it is not advised for long-lasting weight loss because one cap does not fit all.

Why You Don't Need Rapid Weight Loss Diets

The risks of drastic weight loss are enormous - apart from the huge physical demands it creates on the body, there are lots of medical issues that can be traced to it.

People who lose huge amounts of pounds in no time are susceptible to malnutrition, dehydration, electrolyte imbalance, and irritability. Other health issues associated with this type of weight loss are dizziness, constipation, headaches, and fatigue.

In as much as you want to drop those pounds, there is need for common sense - there is no easy route to weight loss. By all means, attack your weight problem in a healthy way to put yourself on the path of success.

Obesity or overweight badly affects the health of a person. To retain the health, it is important to reduce the overweights. A long term weight loss strategy is the best solution to stop being

being overweight.

Losing weight isn't easy but finding the best diet plan for you can make all the difference in the world and I hope to help you with this. It also helps to find healthy substitutes for some of your favorite foods so that you don't feel deprived.

Always ask yourself first if these weight loss programs claiming to be one of the best diet plans will teach you to eat healthily and will you be able to use it for the long term. This is the only way you can maximize the health benefits you are trying to achieve.

CHAPTER 2

SMALL CHANGES EQUAL MASSIVE IMPACT

Sometimes it seems like the only way to lose weight is by adopting a super-strict diet or spending every waking moment at the gym. Luckily, that's not the case. "Healthy, sustainable weight loss is best achieved through small changes to your existing lifestyle. If you want or need to drop pounds, it does take a little effort and consistency.

Rapid weight loss isn't sustainable or healthy for your body, especially if you are in your thirtys. It is much more realistic to rely on a healthy weight loss plan that will provide life-changing results, and easily be sustainable to fit into your life. Healthy weight loss isn't a sprint, it's a marathon. Each pound you lose is another milestone toward your goal, and if done properly, you will permanently keep the weight off for a much more enhanced quality of life.

Here are some tips on how you can lose those unwanted pounds the healthy way:

1. Establish your weight loss goals

Everyone would love to lose 20 pounds in a week - but that is virtually impossible to do healthy way. Make realistic goals for yourself. Goals that are attainable. Be in the mindset that your weight loss goal is for the long term - a life-changing weight loss goal to get and stay healthy for the rest of your life.

Research and find the best weight loss program for you....one that fits into your lifestyle. One that is enjoyable, and adaptable to your life. Then commit and stick to it, and make sure you follow your own set of dieting rules.

2. Kick start your day with breakfast.

Your Mom's old saying is right - breakfast is the most important meal of the day! It will jump-start your metabolism and have you physically and mentally ready to start your day. A healthy breakfast, consisting of lean proteins, low glycemic carbohydrates (whole grain bread, steel-cut oats, etc...), and healthy fats, will give your day a jump start that will boost your metabolism and calorie burn for the rest of the day!

3. Don't "diet".

The key to a healthier way of losing weight is: Eat healthily but don't starve.

The typical weight loss plan has you barely eating, and you may seem happy and feel that you are losing those unwanted inches on your belly and thighs by skipping meals. But remember that this would not last long. Your body cannot tolerate having insufficient food to fuel the energy that you use up every day.

This actually can have the opposite effect. Your body can go into 'starvation mode' and store any food it receives as fat deposits in your body, anticipating a lack of food later.

4. Drink a lot of water.

Proper hydration, preferably through water, is a crucial element in healthy weight loss. Your body needs water not only to operate at peak proficiency but to lose weight - don't worry about fears of gaining 'water weight'.

5. The 'Eat like a bird' meal plan.

Five to six small healthy meals per day is better than three big meals. It evens out your metabolism and keeps it at a high level throughout the day, which keeps your daily caloric burn at a high rate. Additionally, eating frequent, small meals will prevent over-eating - and mentally keep you from feeling that you are 'dieting'.

6. Eat fats, but only the right fats.

Fats are not the devil they have been made out to be in the last 20 years. You need some fats to keep your weight at the proper level. There are such things as healthy fats. Olive, peanut and canola oil have them. Tuna, salmon, and mackerel have omega-3 fats which is good for the heart. Raw almonds and flaxseeds are other fats that are amazing for your body and boost your calorie burning plans.

7. Stay away from simple sugars.

Your meals should be built with a foundation of fruits and vegetables, whole grain bread, rice or whole wheat pasta for those much-needed carbohydrates. Then add some lean proteins and meats. Sweets, sodas, and donuts should be only a rarity in your diet and for an indulgence and reward only.

8. Exercise.

You knew this would be a component. You just can't escape the incredible effects that a good routine exercise program has on your weight loss plan. Not only will it help you melt away the pounds, it will make you feel better, give you more confidence, and keep you energized throughout the day.

Get to the gym, or sign up for exercise classes. If that isn't your thing, here are some other ideas:

- If you only have a few blocks to go, leave your car and walk.
- Instead of taking the elevator, take the stairs.
- Get outdoors and job, or bicycle, or skate.
- Get into sports! Play some basketball with your kids or the neighborhood kids, join a softball team or play racquetball with friends. There are many active things you can do that is fun and exciting.

Use these types of activities, along with your home chores to put some good activity in your life.

It really doesn't matter how much weight you want to lose - the important thing is that you set realistic goals for yourself. Your goals should be attainable, yet doable and sustainable. Go slow.

Once you lost that first 5 or 6 pounds, reward yourself with a good 'cheat' meal, then get back on the program with all the vengeance you had when you started.

Eat frequent healthy meals, drink lots of water, get enough sleep, and stay on your exercise program. You do these things, you will lose weight, and you will be well on your path to a newer, healthier you!

CHAPTER 3 - CHRONO-NUTRITION - A NEW KIND OF DIETARY REGIME

Although new kinds of diets come out on the market every day, weight gain concerns a lot of people. But, results have shown that going from one dietary scheme to another has no real effect after some time, but a harmful yo-yo one. Therefore, rather than following strict and binding regimes where everything is forbidden, why not to opt for a method that teaches you how to eat differently and allows you not to see food as your sworn enemy. This is the chrono-nutrition that has emerged for quite some time and has proved to be effective when adopted as a lifestyle.

It was invented 30 years ago by a French doctor – Alain Delabos. Dr. Alain studied "Chrono Biology". He used his field of study to create this amazing diet.

The science behind this diet lays in the insulin and cortisol levels in the human body as well as digesting enzymes. Controlling how the body uses food nutrients like carbs and fat, insulin is one of the top ranking hormones our body produces. Cortisol, also being one of the main hormones our body produces, controls blood pressure, metabolism rate and other significant functions. Around the clock, each day, the levels of this enzymes and hormones fluctuate.

The Chrono nutrition diet also is known as Chrono diet will allow you to eat everything, and as much as you want. And no, no, no ... no pills... nothing out of the ordinary.

According to this method's followers, you should be able to eat everything. Dieting without limitation, this is the dream of constant weight fighters. It is too good to be true, one might think. In fact, as the name suggests it, this diet refers to eating food (nutrition) at specific times of day (chrono).

The basic principle is rather a simple one: you can eat fatty foods when you get up, hearty dishes at noon (5 hours after the first meal), sugary foods in the afternoon and lighter dishes at bedtime. By precisely following this order, you simply respect the pace of your body. Indeed, as you have noticed yourself, you generally consume more energy in the morning. So it seems unnecessary to eat more at night since you do not need significant calories as sleep does not require high energy expenditure. So if you indulge more calories at dinner, you will just store them unnecessarily.

This idea seems very simple and obvious. Going further into details, you who are a regular of drastic diets will be surprised to learn that it allows the consumption of chocolate, croissants, super sweet cakes, provided they are eaten as a snack, in the afternoon. This would allow you to end the day full of energy provided by the sugar. But if on the contrary, you eat them in the morning, they will be harmful because, at this time of the day, your body really needs fatty foods.

As for meat products, they can be eaten in the morning; all sorts of meat are allowed for lunch and light meats such as chicken can be served for dinner. Carbohydrates are best to be consumed at lunchtime but in small quantities. Eggs (no more than 4 per week) seem particularly recommended especially in the morning or at noon to replace meat. Another difference from other types of regimes is that you cannot eat fruits all day. As they contain sugar, you should try to book them for the afternoon.

By following these principles, you should start losing weight and imposing this regime as a lifestyle will help you permanently stay in shape. When you look closer, you see that all things are allowed, but according to the schedule and you also should be careful not to surpass the total consumption of 1400 kcal a day.

Benefits of Chrono Nutrition

- The advantage of the Chrono nutrition program is that it never occurs so-called "yo-yo" effect (loss – restoring weight), and metabolic disorders are permanently resolved.

- Results showed 100% success with all those who have managed to master the basics of physiological processes.

- The first phase of a program of diet, etc. restrictive regime that lasts 28 days, involves not eating fast (simple) sugars in the form of sweets, fruit, white / yellow sugar, artificial sweeteners, etc., as well as alcoholic beverages containing a high concentration of alcohol, hard drinks. After conducting a restrictive regime, certain products are gradually included in the diet.

- If the patient finds a certain intolerance to a food for a period of 3-6 months is conducted etc. Detoxification of the food, and its implementation, slowly, gradually returning the commodity in the diet.

- Meal timing does play a critical role in determining health outcomes and it can potentially be used as a measure to forestall obesity and other metabolic diseases.

- The Chrono diet isn't demanding that you renounce yourself of food and special food types, all we have to do is to correctly combine groceries in the given time periods.

- Changing some bad habits and adopting healthy eating habits, as well as mastering the basics of the physiology of nutrition will further need to apply permanently in life. And that is the basic principle of chrono nutrition.

Cons of Chrono Nutrition

Some reports have emerged that the Chrono regime is harmful and causes the destruction of the kidneys and that it could have been completed in hospital, and it was revealed that it was a terrible attempt to make an anti-Chrono ad because the pictures from the announcement were not from a hospital but taken from the internet site.

The failure of a company that produces chemicals, ie tablets and weight loss teasers, is over, we do not know how much consumption has fallen, but judging from the attempt to create a false situation (a story), it seems that the situation is bad.

Chrononutrition. Menu For Week And Month

The daily calorie content of dishes should be equal to the daily needs of the person, that is 2000-2200 kcal. Dr. Delabos claims that extra weight will leave through the properly composed menu.

The main recommendations:

- Breakfast should consist of fatty foods – cheese, eggs, ham. The additive may be any vegetable with low starch content. Any fruit, cereal and bread are prohibited. Time for breakfast – 6.30 to 9.30.

- Lunch should include high-protein dishes – fish or chicken breast, vegetable salad of non-starchy vegetables. Time for lunch – 12.00 to 13.30.
- Afternoon snack suggests carbohydrate intake – oatmeal, buckwheat or rice porridge, fruit, chocolate, cocoa. Time for afternoon snack – 17:00 to 18:30.

- Dinner should be light (in the evening the body badly produces enzymes) – a small piece of white fish with vegetables. Time for dinner – after 19.00 (not later than one hour before bedtime).

Let Us Consider The Nutrition Plan of This Method For A Month:

From 2nd to 14th day

During this period it is recommended to eat low-calorie foods, but at the same time ensure that your menu is the most well-balanced. This is necessary because at this time the level of the hormone ghrelin in the female body is significantly reduced.

From 15th to 21st day of the cycle

At this time, the excess liquid can be delayed in the body. It is recommended to reduce the intake of carbohydrates – refuse sweets and a large amount of fruit (it will help the process of weight loss). At the same time, you should increase the number of proteins in the menu – meat and fatty acids omega-3.

From 22nd to 28th day

You may feel a sharp appetite increase. In order to maintain the normal weight and prevent overeating, you need to increase the daily caloric intake to 1600 kcal. It is also recommended additionally to start taking drugs containing magnesium and iron.

The Approximate Menu For A Week:

Monday

- Breakfast: 100 grams of cheese, 70 grams of bread from coarse grinding, 20 grams of butter, tea or coffee without sugar.

- Lunch: two cutlets of chicken or turkey, vegetable risotto.

- Snack: 30 grams of dark chocolate, fruit or berries to your taste, tea or coffee (maybe with sugar).

- Dinner: baked sea fish, vegetable salad.

Tuesday

- Breakfast: omelette or two fried eggs, toast with cheese, coffee or tea without sugar.

- Lunch: salad of seafood and fresh vegetables, boiled rice.

- Snack: nuts, 2 scoops of ice cream or sorbet, tea or coffee (maybe with sugar).

- Dinner: salad of beans with the addition of a handful of cashew nuts.

Wednesday

- Breakfast: 2 hard-boiled eggs, toast with cheese, tea or coffee without sugar.

- Lunch: boiled beef, salad from fresh vegetables.

- Snack: a handful of nuts, a glass of freshly squeezed juice (any fruit of your choice).

- Dinner: boiled rice with a salad of fresh vegetables and grated cheese.

Thursday

- Breakfast: 100 grams of cheese, 70 grams of solid types of bread, 20 grams of butter, tea or coffee without sugar.

- Lunch: mashed potatoes, two chicken cutlets.

- Snack: 80 grams of any pie, tea or coffee (maybe with sugar).

- Dinner: boiled asparagus dressed with lemon juice with olive oil.

Friday

- Breakfast: omelette with two eggs, a tomato, toast with cheese, tea or coffee without sugar.

- Lunch: barley porridge with the addition of mushrooms.

- Snack: baked apple with cinnamon and honey, a glass of freshly squeezed fruit juice to your choice.

- Dinner: grilled vegetables.

Saturday

- Breakfast: 1-2 middle boiled eggs, toast with avocado and tomato, tea or coffee without sugar.

- Lunch: tomato soup with meatballs of beef.

- Snack: 80 grams of ice cream, tea or coffee (maybe with sugar).

- Dinner: squids, steamed with vegetables.

Sunday

- Breakfast: 100 grams of hard cheese, 70 grams of bread from coarse grinding, 20 grams of butter, tea or coffee without sugar.

- Lunch: millet porridge with the addition of pumpkin.

- Snack: 30 grams of dark chocolate, two fruit to your taste, tea or coffee (maybe with sugar).

- Dinner: salmon fillet with lemon juice, squash caviar.

Once your body gets used to the chrono-nutrition diet you won't even know that you are "always being careful" what you eat or combine. You will have more energy during the day and sleep better at night. Chrono nutrition diet is not a diet, it is a way of life. And many that practice it have shown that it is not hard, but only healthy and better than what others do

CHAPTER 4 -LOW CARB DIET

What Is a Low Carb Diet?

The term "low carb diet" is a broad term, and its principals have been incorporated into numerous different diet plans, including the Atkins, South Beach, and the Zone diet. In its most basic definition, a low carb diet is one that limits a participant's consumption of foods that are high in carbohydrates. The diet may be best explained by the "No White Foods" approach. A simple approach to establishing a low carbohydrates diet, it means that an individual must eliminate sugars, white flour, white rice, and potatoes from their diet to lose weight.

It is common for some individuals to mistake the low carbohydrates diet with the low carb phase of some popular diets, like Induction phase of the Atkins diet. Low carb phases of such diets are designed to last only for short periods of time, and more carbohydrates are gradually phased into the diet after the phase has passed. However, technically defined, any diet that focuses on the reduction of carbohydrates is considered. The mainstream recommendation is for an individual's diet to consist of 50-65% of their calories coming from carbohydrates. However, a diet where less than 40% of the individual's calories are coming from carbohydrates is generally considered low carb.

In clinical trials and studies, low carb diets have been proven effective in inducing weight loss for up to one year. After this point, the effectiveness of a low carb diet begins to wear off. A similar 2007 JAMA study revealed that obese women who followed a low carbohydrates diet for twelve months fared better in terms of weight loss and overall health than their obese counterparts who followed the Zone, Ornish, or learn diets. Another unauthenticated study examined the lives of 100,000 individuals over 20 years. Those who followed the diet faithfully lived an average of 2.8 years longer than their counterparts.

Although there are numerous diets to choose from, almost all of them cut sugars and starches out of one's diet. If an individual is interested in participating in a low carb diet, then their first step should be to visit their primary care physician. There are numerous false myths floating around, and a medical professional will be able to dispel fact from fiction, as well as assist the patient in devising the effective low carbs for their unique body.

Annoying Low Carb Diet Myths
The low carb diet brings in some criticism and some unfounded MYTHS due to its enormous success. We'll hope to have eradicated all these unwarranted notions from your mind by the time you finish reading this article in its entirety.

Here are the most common myths associated with the low carb

diet plan. They're not in any particular order so, don't read anything to this:

1. The fact Dr Atkins died, people also pronounced dead it low carb diet plan, the famous "Atkins diet" - obviously named after him since he was the founder of the plan, for those of you that didn't know this. Dr Atkins actually died of brain injuries resulting from a fall, and this has absolutely nothing whatsoever to do with the diet he famously founded.

2. It has been said that the low carb diet will reduce the amount of calcium in your body. This couldn't be farther from the truth, as since the low carb diet is rich in protein, this in fact actually prevents calcium from entering your urine.

3. They say the low carb diet plan will damage one's kidney. Not unless one already has a kidney defect, because the low carb diet, though rich in protein, this is not what the entire meal is made of. Once on low carb diet, one still must observe the balancing of the meal consumed. It has been said that some Doctors actually recommend the low carb diet for some of their patients in other to treat kidney problems. As I'm not a doctor, I

always and shall continue to encourage people wanting to lose weight to seek professional advice before embarking on any form of weight loss or diet programs or plan.

4. Moving from kidney, there's also this myth that whilst on low carb diet, that you're dicing with heart disease. To the contrary, it's a fact that the low carb diet plan actually reduces the risk of having a heart disease. It has also been proven that even food containing lots of animal fat and proteins do not constitute a risk for heart disease.

5. There is no fibre present in the low carb diet. The low carb diet is, on the contrary, full of fibre, and research also shows that the presence of this fibre actually lessens the effect and the amount of carbohydrate in one's body. Which makes the low carb diet a very pragmatic diet plan?

6. Whilst on low carb diet, you're not allowed fruits or vegetables. This one actually gets me mad, because it's not a secret that the population for one reason or another do just not like eating fruits and vegetables. This goes back for years, and the Governments all over the world are now making it a point of duty by recommending the

daily intakes. So, just because people have preferences doesn't mean it's down to the low carb diet plan.

7. Low carb diet means total elimination of carbohydrate. Even the most critical doctors, scientists, or nutritionists will dispel this, as in any given meal, one must have at least 45% - 65% carbohydrates in their meals, depending on each individual, of course.

8. Low carb diets will attract permanent bad breath. This to some extent is true, but not because you're on low carb diet plan. This is simply because, people, regardless of what weight loss or diet program the embark on, they feel they have to abstain from other meals such as eating fruits and vegetables. Even if one's not on any form of diet, by not eating fruits and vegetables will certainly attract bad breath. To combat this is simple, just eat more fruits and vegetables on a daily basis. This has nothing to do with low carb diet alone!

Low Carb Diet Meal prep

Having many low carb recipes at your disposal is essential if you are going to seriously do a low carb diet. It'd be a step even better if you could compile all the recipes that you have a book - your very own low carb recipe book with your favourite recipes

As a busy woman, I know how hard it is to find the time to cook but once you found some simple recipes that you can also prepare for the other members of the family it's going to become a habit to eat healthy.

One of my favourite websites when preparing low carb meals is www.dietdoctor.com. By having a low carb recipe book, you will soon see how it can make life easier since you don't have to try coming up with different recipes for your meal every day. People are creatures of habits, so you wil probably end up repeating the recipes bi-weekly or monthly.

Benefits of Low Carb Diet

Low-Carb Diets Kill Your Appetite (in a Good Way)

Hunger is the single worst side effect of dieting. It is one of the main reasons why many people feel miserable and eventually give up on their diets.One of the best things about eating low-carb is that it leads to an automatic reduction in appetite

Low-Carb Diets Lead to More Weight Loss

Cutting carbs is one of the simplest and most effective ways to lose weight. Studies show that people on low-carb diets lose more weight, faster, than people on low-fat diets... even when the low-fat dieter's are actively restricting calories.

One of the reasons for this is that low-carb diets tend to get rid of excess water from the body. Because they lower insulin levels, the kidneys start shedding excess sodium, leading to rapid weight loss in the first week or two

Helps Fat loss from The Abdominal Cavity

It's where that fat is stored that determines how it will affect our health and risk of disease.

Most importantly, we have subcutaneous fat (under the skin) and then we have visceral fat (in the abdominal cavity).Visceral fat is fat that tends to lodge around the organs.

Having a lot of fat in that area can drive inflammation, insulin resistance and is believed to be a leading driver of the metabolic dysfunction that is so common in Western countries today (

Low-carb diets are very effective at reducing the harmful abdominal fat.

Not only do they cause more fat loss than low-fat diets, an even greater proportion of that fat is coming from the abdominal cavity.

Over time, this should lead to a drastically reduced risk of heart disease and type 2 diabetes.

Blood Pressure Tends to Go Down

Having elevated blood pressure (hypertension) is an important risk factor for many diseases. This includes heart disease, stroke, kidney failure and many others. Low-carb diets are an effective way to reduce blood pressure, which should lead to a reduced risk of these diseases and help you live longer

Low-Carb Diets Improve The Pattern of LDL Cholesterol

Low-density lipoprotein (LDL) is often referred to as the "bad" cholesterol (again, it is actually a protein). It is known that people who have high LDL are much more likely to have heart attacks. However... What scientists have now learned is that the type of LDL matters. Not all of them are equal.

In this regard, the size of the particles is important. People who have mostly small particles have a high risk of heart disease, while people who have mostly large particles have a low risk.

It turns out that low-carb diets actually turn the LDL particles from small to large while reducing the number of LDL particles floating around in the bloodstream

Cons of Low Carb Diets

General Body Weakness

When you make a transition from a crab-dependent diet to a

low-carb diet, your body needs to adjust to the changes, according to Becky Hand, a licensed and registered dietitian. Low-carb diets cause lack of energy in your body because carbohydrates play a role in the burning of fats, which produce energy. Lack of energy in your body can cause dizziness, nausea, headaches and fatigue.

Bad Breath

Low-carb diets lead to incomplete burning of fats to produce energy in your body, and in the process, ketones are produced, says Anssi H Manninen, an exercise physiologist specializing in sports nutrition and ergogenic aids. Excess ketones in your body come out through your urine and saliva. This causes bad breath among people on low-carb diets. Though you cannot do much to stop bad breath, drinking water and chewing sugar-free gum can help you suppress bad breath, says Shannon Clark, a certified personal trainer and author of "8 Low-Carb Conundrums."

Constipation

Foods in low-carb diets such as beef have little fibre and cause reduction in body fibre, which can lead to constipation. However, constipation occurs due to lack of roughage in your body regardless your nutrition plan, says Clark. You can avoid constipation by including vegetables in your diet since they have soluble fibre that slows the movement of food in the intestines to ensure complete digestion of food.

Dehydration

Low-carb diets burn glycogen stores in your body, which have water. Excretion of ketones through your urine causes frequent urination. This loss of water leads to dehydration when you are on a low-carb diet. Dehydration leads to headaches and fatigue. Take a lot of water to replenish the lost water as a remedy to dehydration caused by low-carb diet, reports the Mayo Clinic.

Muscle Cramps

Diets low in carbohydrates have an effect on your muscles. This is caused by the dehydration due to your low-carb diet and lack of vitamins that are important for the well-being of your muscles. Muscle cramps reduce your fitness and energy levels, says Doctor Arne Astrup. Consume fruits and vegetables with essential vitamins as a remedy for muscle cramps.

CHAPTER 5 - INTERMITTENT FASTING

Intermittent fasting (also referred to as I.F.) has become quite the phenomenon these days. Recent studies showed that people who tried it have lost weight increased health, and believed to have a long lifespan. Basically, intermittent fasting is a pattern of eating that alternates between periods of fasting, usually consuming only water, and non-fasting, usually eating anything a person wants no matter how fattening. In other words, a person can eat anything he wants during a 24-hour period and fast for the next 24 hours. This approach to weight control seems to be supported by science, as well as religious and cultural practices around the globe. Adherents of intermittent fasting claim that this practice is a way to become more circumspect about food.

Martin Berkhan is the guy who many mistakenly believe started the whole movement of intermittent fasting.

Although he wasn't the first on the scene, he probably made the biggest impact on the internet. Just a couple of years after starting his site, tens of thousands of readers were hitting his site each day!

Martin's method of intermittent fasting is to reduce the time eating to an 8 window. You wind up fasting for 16 hours and are allowed to eat in an 8 hour time period.

Advantages Of Intermittent Fasting

1. **Counting Calories Is Unnecessary On Intermittent Fasting:** Almost all dietary approaches involve counting calories. While this may be necessary following these short-term eating plans, it is almost impossible to do this long-term. This means that when the "diet" is over, the classical rebound fat gain is just around the corner after a period of rigidly controlling all food.

2. **You Don't Have To Go Hungry On Intermittent Fasting:** When you are eating all your daily calories in a window of several hours, it becomes much more difficult to overeat when compared to a traditional grazing approach. If you are fasting, you are not worrying about whether a snack is okay or not. Fasting is not eating and when you break the fast, you eat if you are hungry. Simple!

3. **Your Body Doesn't Try To Hang On To Its Fat Stores When Intermittent Fasting:** Most dietary approaches are necessarily restrictive. Your body is permanently deprived of enough food and reacts be going into starvation mode. It hangs on to all your fat stores and slows down your metabolism, exactly the opposite of what we want. However, when you can eat satisfaction

as is the case on a fasting diet, your body responds by continuing to drop body fat.

4. **An Intermittent Fasting Diet Is Less Restrictive Than Other Diets**: Let's be clear here if your idea of good food is a burger and fries, nothing is going to help you until you change your perception. However, it is perfectly possible and even helpful to have some leeway in what you eat. Sure, start with your protein and veggies, but some of what you like has some interesting and positive hormonal effects if you are trying to get lean or even build some muscle.

5. **An Intermittent Fasting Diet Adapts To You**: This is the real beauty of this approach. Instead of trying to find exactly the right number of grams of carbs or whatever at 10 am, you fit your daily fast to your life and goals. Some find a 16 hour fast from evening until the next day at lunchtime works best. Others prefer a 24-hour cycle or even a 4-hour eating window. All of these are possible and have different advantages. It is a lifestyle rather than a diet.

Types of Intermittent Fasting

There are many different popular intermittent fasts and hundreds more possible variations. There are four kinds of intermittent fasts that are most basic and frequently used.

The 16/8 Method: Fast For 16 Hours Each Day.

The 16/8 Method involves fasting every day for 14-16 hours and restricting your daily "eating window" to 8-10 hours.

Within the eating window, you can fit in 2, 3 or more meals.

This method is also known as the Leangains protocol and was popularized by fitness expert Martin Berkhan.

Doing this method of fasting can actually be as simple as not eating anything after dinner, and skipping breakfast.

For example, if you finish your last meal at 8 pm and then don't eat until 12 noon the next day, then you are technically fasting for 16 hours between meals.

It is very important to eat mostly healthy foods during your eating window. This won't work if you eat lots of junk food or excessive amounts of calories.

Benefits of Intermittent Fasting 16:8?

Increased Fat Loss

IF can help you to get exceptionally lean, and shift stubborn fat once you already have a fairly low body fat percentage, in the low to mid-teens. Those with a higher body fat percentage will also see more significant weight loss whilst following IF, and often will see results after only a short period of committing to the protocol.

Less Cravings

In addition to the increased rate of fat loss, IF prevents you from craving unhealthy food. It teaches you when you are physically hungry, and when you just fancy something to eat. It acts as a hunger suppressant; and you will find that you will be more satisfied following a meal.

Improved Insulin Response

After fasting for the 16 hour period, when you do eventually break the fast, you will be more sensitive to insulin, and therefore your insulin levels will be more stable and fluctuate less. It also means an improved rate of protein synthesis, since insulin is a powerful hormone for controlling the rate of it. The improved insulin response contributes to the fact you will have less cravings and appreciate your food more.

Improved Cognitive Function

One of the main worries before trying IF was getiigntired and sluggish in the morning. You'll found that in fact when in a fasted state, you felt better and performed better. Since blood is not being pumped to your digestive system, as it normally would after a meal, more oxygen is sent to other parts of your body e.g. muscles during a workout or your brain.

Improved Overall Health

Studies have shown that IF can lead to a longer life, and also reduce the risk of cancer. It helps to cleanse your body and give your internal organs a break.

The 5:2 Diet: Fast For 2 Days Per Week.

The 5:2 diet involves eating normally 5 days of the week while restricting calories to 500-600 on two days of the week.

This diet is also called the Fast diet. On the fasting days, it is recommended that women eat 500 calories, and men 600 calories.

For example, you might eat normally on all days except Mondays and Thursdays, where you eat two small meals (250 calories per meal for women, and 300 for men).

There is no rule as to what or when you must eat on the fasting days.

Generally, there are two meal patterns that people use:

- Three small meals: Usually breakfast, lunch and dinner.

- Two slightly bigger meals: Only lunch and dinner.

Here Are A Few Examples Of Foods That May Be Suitable For Fast Days:

- A generous portion of vegetables.

- Natural yoghurt with berries.

- Boiled or baked eggs.

- Grilled fish or lean meat.

- Cauliflower rice.

- Soups (for example miso, tomato, cauliflower or vegetable).

- Low-calorie cup soups.

- Black coffee.

- Tea.

- Still or sparkling water.

Eat-Stop-Eat: Do A 24-Hour Fast, Once Or Twice A Week.

Eat-Stop-Eat involves a 24-hour fast, either once or twice per week.

This method was popularized by fitness expert Brad Pilon and has been quite popular for a few years.

Eat Stop Eat works in a fairly simple way: You fast once or twice a week, aiming for a complete break from food for 24 hours at a time. For example, you might eat normally until 7 p.m. on a Saturday, then fast until 7 p.m. on Sunday, resuming regular eating at that time. If you can't make it the full 24 hours,

20 to 24 hours will also work. For the next couple of days, eat approximately 2,000 calories a day for women and 2,500 for men; never fast on consecutive days. After several normal eating days, you can have another fast and repeat the schedule. Do not exceed two fasts in any one week. By doing even one fast a week, will create a calorie deficit of 10 percent.

The Warrior Diet

If you are one of those people who hate eating breakfast and find it much more convenient and enjoyable to eat one large meal rather than several small meals a day then you will not find the Warrior diet interesting but very enjoyable. The diet is based on the habits of ancient warriors who in preparing for battle ate little during the day but enjoyed a huge meal at night when they were less likely to be attacked and therefore could rest and enjoy their food.

Rather than a diet, it is a more an overall fitness program that combines diet, exercise and sound nutrition in a kind of feast or famine arrangement. The idea behind the diet is that during the day when you should be most active you should eat very little. Eating a very small amount of food with no or limited protein stresses the body making you burn calories faster and adds to mental alertness.

Step #1

The first step has to do with your mindset. This actually holds true for every single diet out there, and there are way too many to name. To lose weight easily and effectively, you have to make it one of your primary goals. Losing weight for your own personal reasons is always better than trying to do it for someone else.

The majority of people start eating healthy and exercising in order to please others. Some train with the intention of attracting a potential mate, while others do it because getting compliments on their appearance gives them an ego boost. Neither one of these situations works very well for long-term success. Sticking to a diet and exercise program is much easier when you decide to do it for yourself, and forget everyone else.

Step #2

The second step to making this diet a success is eating your biggest meal at night. This one is tough to get used to for some people because it goes against everything you've been told to do before. Having either three large meals per day or six smaller ones are the most common eating schedules.

I hate to say it, but this diet will not work for you if you skip this important step. By skipping the big breakfast and lunch, and having your largest meal in the evening, you will become leaner and stronger. The best news is that you can see and feel these benefits without having to alter the number of calories that you consume.

Step #3

The third success step has to do with the foods you decide to put into your body. If you constantly eat whatever you feel like eating, you will be very disappointed with your results. This isn't exclusive to the Warrior Diet. It applies to every single diet out there. Fast food is what you should pay the most attention to.

Eating fast food on a regular basis does absolutely nothing to help you lose weight. It is very high in fat, and the majority of the calories are empty (do not provide nutritional value for your body). Stick to the healthy stuff instead: fresh fruit and vegetables, nuts, eggs, fish, and low-fat dairy products. These foods are much better for you because they contain calories that can actually be used for energy.

Step #4

The fourth and final step deals with the time of day you decide to exercise. To achieve the best possible results, make sure you exercise during the under-eating phase. You might be thinking that doing this will make you weak, but combining exercise with under-eating actually helps you resist fatigue.

To Wrap Things Up... Let's go through the steps one more time. First, you have to make up your own mind about wanting to lose weight. Second, make sure to eat your biggest meal in the evening. Third, keep an eye on what you eat. Fourth, try to exercise during the under-eating phase.

CHAPTER 6 - ADAPTING AND STICKING TO THE DIET

It is quite common for people to begin a weight loss program at the start of the New Year. After days of merrymaking and partying during the holidays, people are often scrambling to lose the bulge that seemed to develop after several cups of eggnog and pieces of gingerbread cookies. However, after a few visits to the gym or several days of dieting, many people's interest in going ahead with losing weight tend to wane.

If you are one of the people who are starting to lose interest in shedding off the pounds that you have gained during the holidays or even throughout all these years, you probably need to set concrete goals of what you want to happen. After knowing what you want to achieve, say lose 10 pounds in 3 months, you need a little bit of motivation to push you to continue with your diet plan and exercise regimen.

Here are some of the things that can encourage you to stick with the program and lose that excess weight:

Announce Your Target Weight Loss To Others

If you are a competitive person, you need to tell your family and friends about your weight loss plan so that you will feel a little motivated to stick to your exercise and diet regimen. Since you have already told other people of your specific goals, you will have to work hard to achieve them. You will have bragging rights, so to speak, if you actually show your friends that you have the discipline and the will to really realize your dreams.

Another reason why you need to tell your friends and family about your weight loss plan is for support. If you are overweight or obese for a long time, your family and close friends will be more than happy to help you with your goals. They are the people who want you to be healthy and have confidence in the way you look. So when you are out for a dinner, they will be there to remind you to skip the refillable sodas or sugar-rich mud pie.

Be Constantly Reminded Of Your Goal

In order for the idea of shedding pounds to sink into your subconscious, you need to be constantly reminded of how you want to look and what you want to weigh. Thus, put pictures of people who have the ideal weight you are pining for on your refrigerator's door, your kitchen counter and even on your bedside table. Some people even put such pictures in their wallets so that every time they get money to buy a chocolate bar, they are reminded that this bar puts them farther away from what they want to look like.

Find A Partner

The chance for success is higher if you have a partner in losing weight. You can find a partner in another friend who is also suffering from the bulge, a spouse who has a big belly, or even a brother, sister or parent who also needs to be fit. Sometimes you cannot count on discipline alone to push you to go to the gym or exercise. The buddy system will prevent procrastination and laziness. Furthermore, it is much more fun to workout while talking with friends.

Hang That Dress

Splurge on a to-die-for dress that is a few dress sizes smaller. Then, hang it in your bedroom so that you will be able to see it when you wake up and go to sleep. This dress will motivate you to keep on moving and to skip junk foods for a midnight snack.

Reward Yourself –

The hardest part about dieting or just trying to eat healthily is sticking to your good intentions. How can you stick to it without all the heartache? Simply learn to reward yourself. We are just like children if you keep saying no, eventually you are going to cave in. It is important to reward yourself for good behavior. Why not pick one day during the week as your "cheat" day where you can choose one thing to eat that you have been craving that is not part of your diet? Then, if you are good all week, you can have your reward. It really helps to keep you on your diet and keep you consistent.

CONCLUSION

If you want to be successful in any diet, whether for weight loss or health reasons, the key is to stick to the diet. Although this can seem daunting at times, you can be successful if you are reasonable in your food and exercise choices, if you plan ahead, and if you learn to reward yourself. Yes, you can be healthy and fit forever, just remember that the most important characteristic of most suffesfull people is persistence, that's the only way you can achiever what you want.

If you have enjoied this bookand you are planning to implement the change to your lifestyle, please recommend it to a friend and leave a review if you are not too busy. This will make the book easier to find by other women.

Thank you for reading this book. If you have enjoyed this book please click on the link to leave a review.

ABOUT THE AUTHOR

Roxana is a Secondary Mathics teacher based in London. She has a Master's in Science and is passionate about research and education. Roxana enjoys learning new things and sharing her knewledge on different topics, including weight loss.